The Let's Talk Library™

Let's Talk About
Needing Glasses

Diane Shaughnessy

The Rosen Publishing Group's
PowerKids Press™
New York

Published in 1997 by The Rosen Publishing Group, Inc.
29 East 21st Street, New York, NY 10010

First Edition

Book Design: Erin McKenna

Photo Illustrations: Cover © Bill Tucker/International Stock; p. 7 © Eric Berndt/Midwestock; all other photo illustrations by Maria Moreno.

Shaughnessy, Diane.
    Let's talk about needing glasses / Diane Shaughnessy.
        p.   cm. — (The let's talk library)
    Includes index.
    Summary: Discusses some reasons why people need to wear glasses, with steps in getting glasses, the teasing one sometimes receives with a change in looks, and the possibility that glasses occasionally break.
    ISBN 0-8239-5042-5
    1. Eyeglasses—Juvenile literature. 2. Vision disorders—Juvenile literature. [1. Eyeglasses.] I. Title.   II. Series.
    RE976.S53 1996
    617.7'522—dc20   96-41651
                                                                              CIP
                                                                              AC

Manufactured in the United States of America

Table of Contents

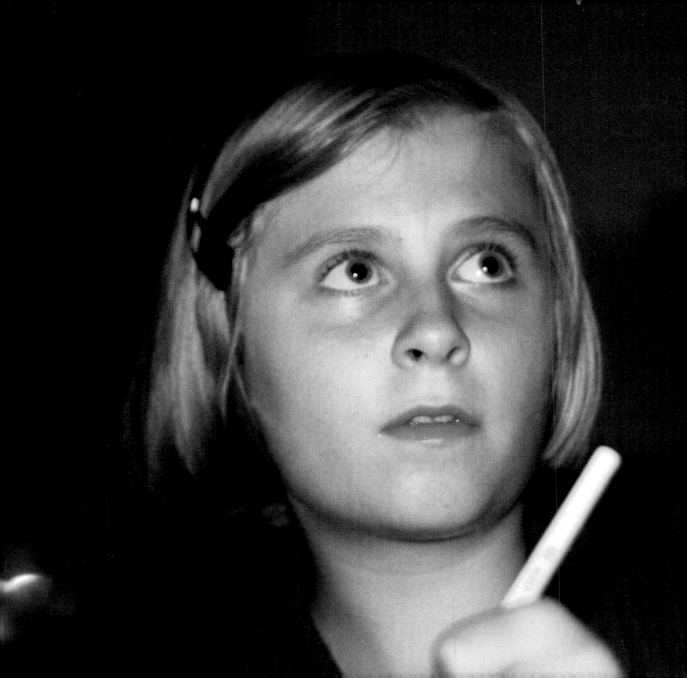

Fuzzy Edges

Billie's teacher asked her to read aloud from her book. Billie could see all of the words. She read them very well. Then the teacher asked Billie to read the words on the blackboard. But those words had fuzzy edges. Billie tried harder, but she still couldn't see them well. She tried guessing, but the teacher knew something was wrong. He asked Billie to read the blackboard from the front row. Now Billie could see the words clearly. The teacher told Billie that she may need to wear glasses.

◀ If you have trouble reading the blackboard, you may need glasses.

Needing Glasses

Some people have good **vision** (VIH-zhun). They can see both far away and close up. But some people have a hard time seeing things clearly. They have poor vision. But they can wear glasses to help them see better. People who wear glasses often see better than people who don't wear glasses. Their glasses make their vision much better.

Wearing glasses helps people see more clearly. ▶

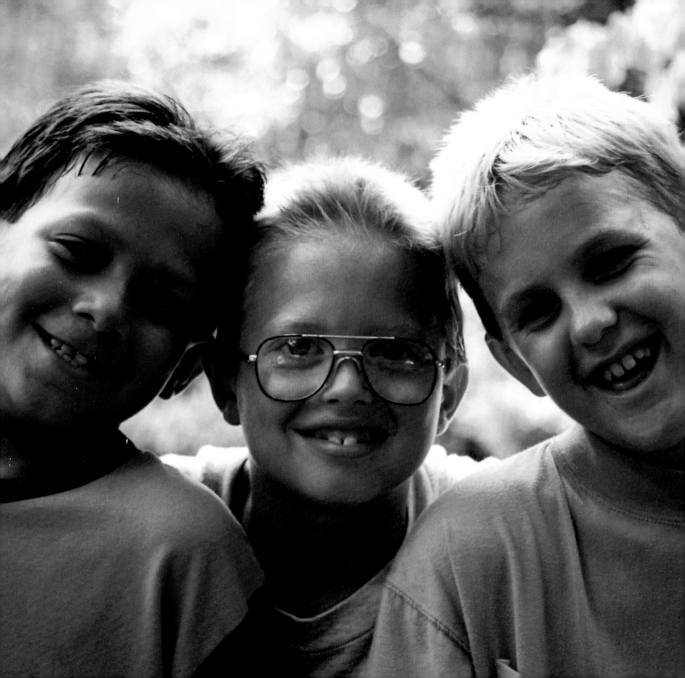

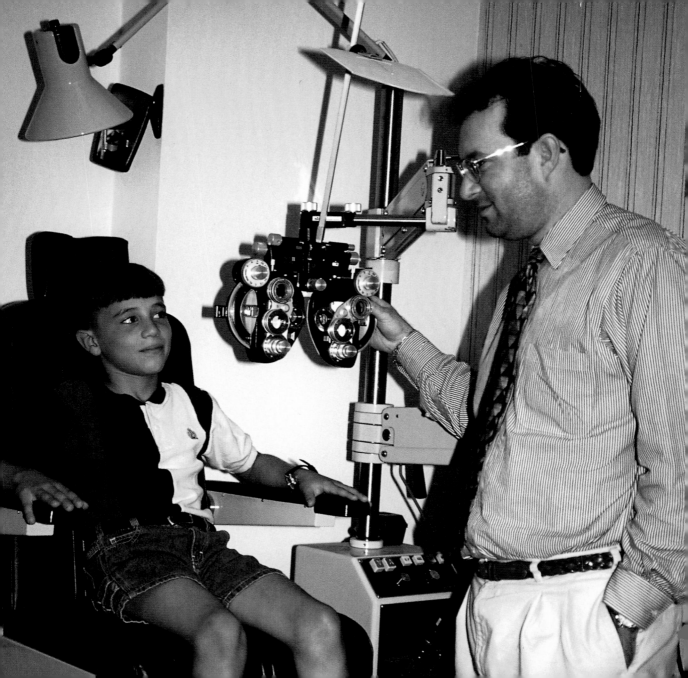

Going to the Eye Doctor

If you have a hard time seeing clearly, your mom or dad may take you to the **optometrist** (op-TOM-ih-trist). An optometrist is an eye doctor. First he will put special drops in your eyes. They may make your vision **blurry** (BLUR-ee), but they help the doctor **examine** (eg-ZAM-in) your eyes. He may have you look through a machine. He may also ask you to read letters from a chart on the wall. All of these things help the optometrist learn what kind of vision you have and what kind of glasses you may need.

◀ The machine that you look through may seem scary, but it doesn't hurt at all.

Being Nearsighted

People who can see things that are near them are **nearsighted** (NEER-sy-tid). A person who is nearsighted can see the words in books clearly. But she can't see clearly things that are far away from her. She may have a hard time watching a movie or seeing someone who waves to her from the other side of the street. Billie, the girl at the beginning of this book, is nearsighted.

A person who is nearsighted needs glasses ▶
to see things that are far away.

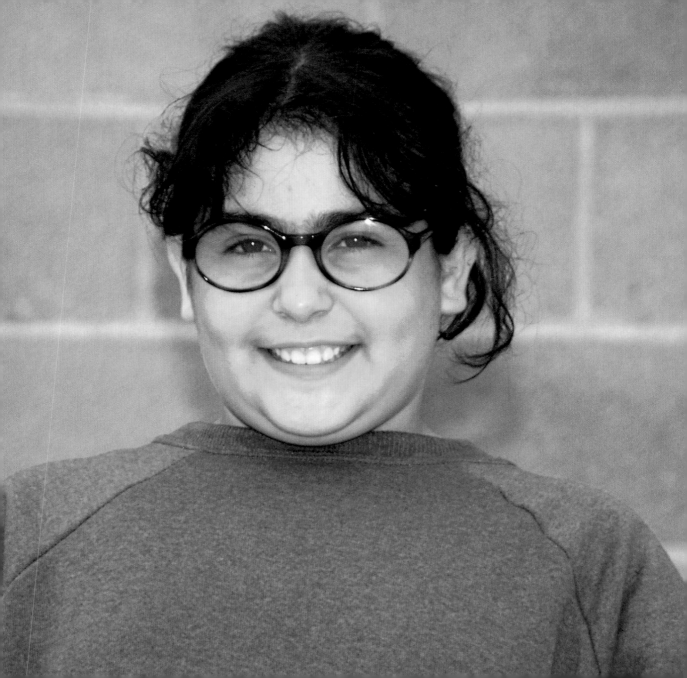

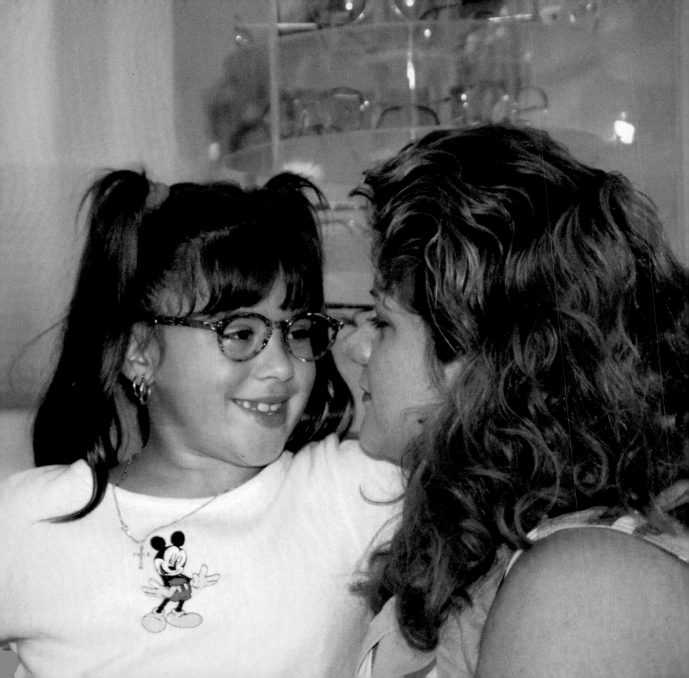

Being Farsighted

People who can see things that are far away are **farsighted** (FAR-sy-tid). A person who is farsighted can see a score at a baseball game easily. But she can't see things that are close to her. She may have trouble seeing the pieces of a puzzle that are right in front of her.

◀ A person who is farsighted needs glasses to see things or people that are up close.

Getting Glasses

The optometrist will write out a **prescription** (preh-SCRIP-shun) for glasses. Your mom or dad will take that prescription to the **optician** (op-TIH-shun), the person who makes the glasses. Glasses are made of glass or plastic **lenses** (LEN-zes) and frames. The optician will make the lenses. You and your parents will choose a pair of frames. Frames come in many different colors and styles. You can choose a pair that you like and that is **comfortable** (KUMF-ter-bul) to wear. You may even be able to pick out a case for your glasses.

It is important that your glasses are comfortable to wear. ▶

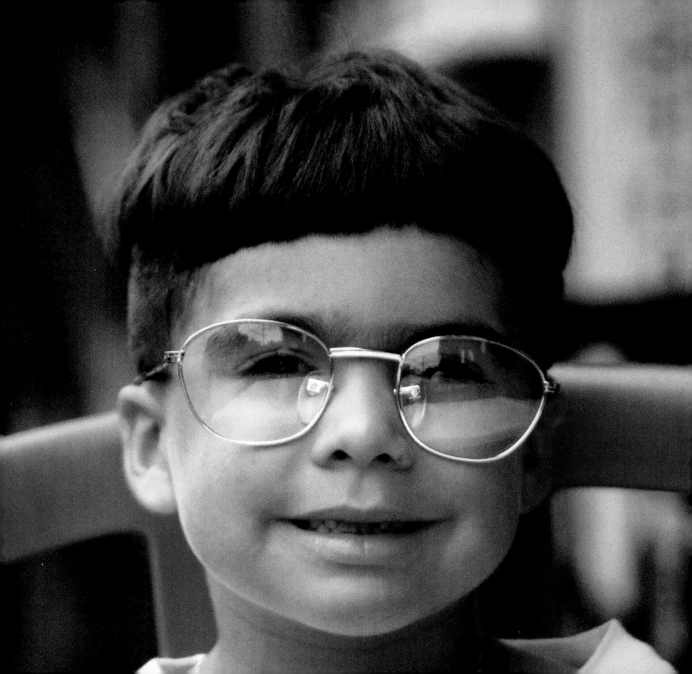

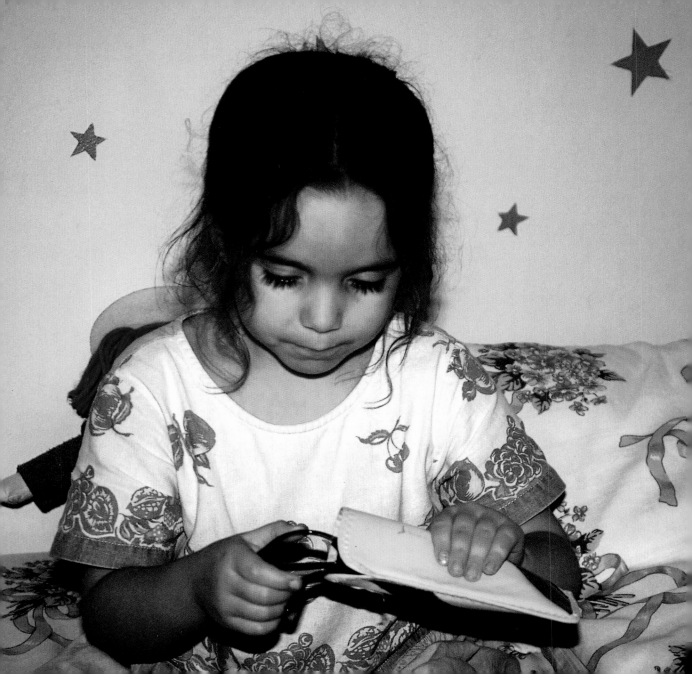

Your First Pair of Glasses

In about a week, you will have a new pair of glasses. You will be amazed at how clearly you can see! You may not have to wear your glasses all the time. It's a good idea to put your glasses in their case whenever you take them off. The optician will give you a soft cloth and a special lens cleaner. She will show you how to clean your glasses. The cleaner you keep your glasses, the better you will be able to see.

◀ The best way to keep your glasses safe is to put them in their case whenever you take them off.

When to Wear Your Glasses

The optician will tell you when you need to wear your glasses. Some people need to wear them all the time. Others don't. If you are nearsighted, you will need to wear them when you are looking at things that are far away. You will need them to read the blackboard at school. If you are farsighted, you will need to wear your glasses when you read a book or play a board game. It is a good idea to carry your glasses with you all the time. You never know when you might need them!

Someone who is farsighted will need to wear his glasses when he reads. ▶

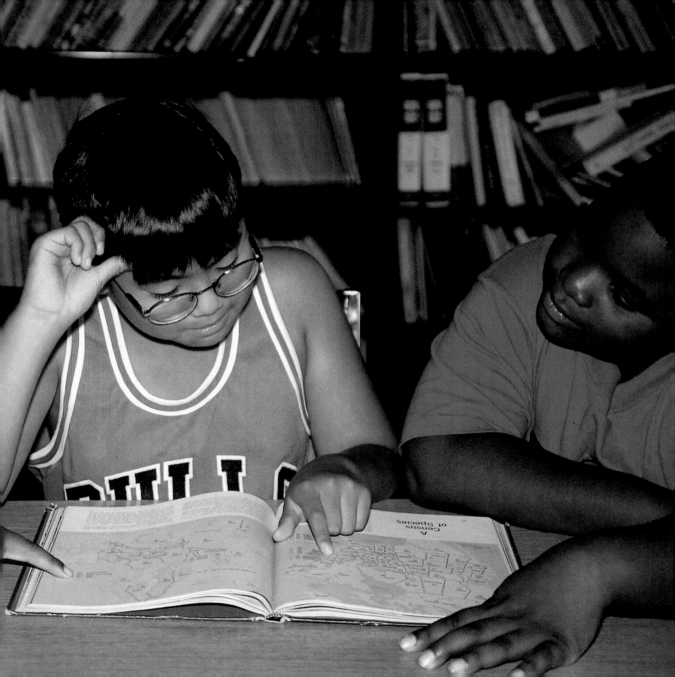

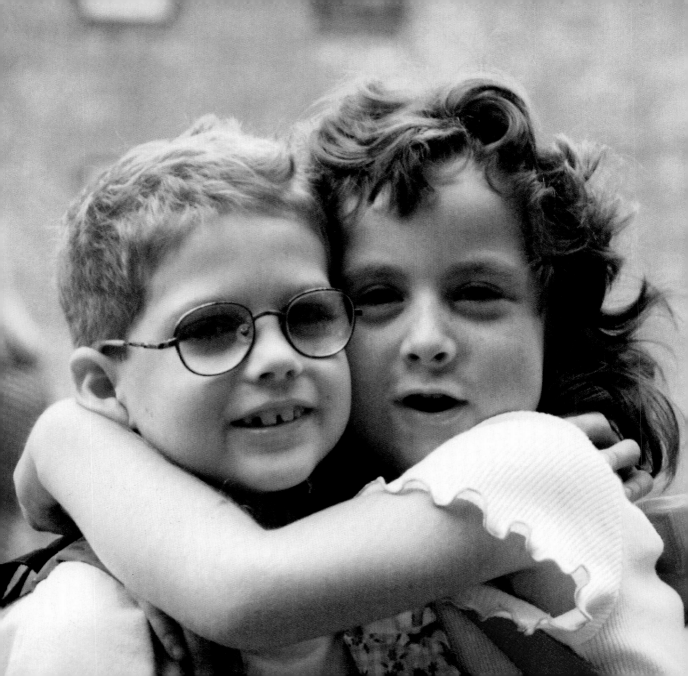

Showing Your Friends

You may know other kids who wear glasses. You may have heard people **tease** (TEEZ) them or call them names such as "four-eyes." You may be afraid that people will tease you or call you names. And they may. People can be mean sometimes. But you don't have to let them hurt your feelings. You can walk away. Or you can say something like, "Now I can see you better." People will get used to seeing you with glasses. They'll stop saying mean things. And you will be proud that you are able to see better.

21

◀ Your friends will get used to seeing you with glasses.

Oops! New Glasses

Even if you are very careful, your glasses may break. You may leave them on the floor and step on them. Or you may break them playing a sport. You may lose them. These things happen to most people. Don't be afraid to tell your mom or dad. They might be upset or angry for a little while. But they will be glad that you told them. It is important to them that you see well. Your mom or dad will get your glasses fixed or get you new ones. But it is up to you to take good care of them.

Glossary

blurry (BLUR-ee) Not clear.

comfortable (KUMF-ter-bul) Feeling relaxed; having no pain.

examine (eg-ZAM-in) Look at someone or something closely.

farsighted (FAR-sy-tid) Seeing distant things more clearly than near ones.

lens (LENZ) Curved piece of glass or plastic that helps a person see more clearly.

nearsighted (NEER-sy-tid) Seeing near things more clearly than distant ones.

optician (op-TIH-shun) Maker or seller of glasses.

optometrist (op-TOM-ih-trist) Person who is trained to examine eyes and prescribe glasses.

prescription (preh-SCRIP-shun) Written order for preparing glasses or medicine.

tease (TEEZ) To make fun of someone by telling jokes or name-calling.

vision (VIH-zhun) Sight.

Index